I0114983

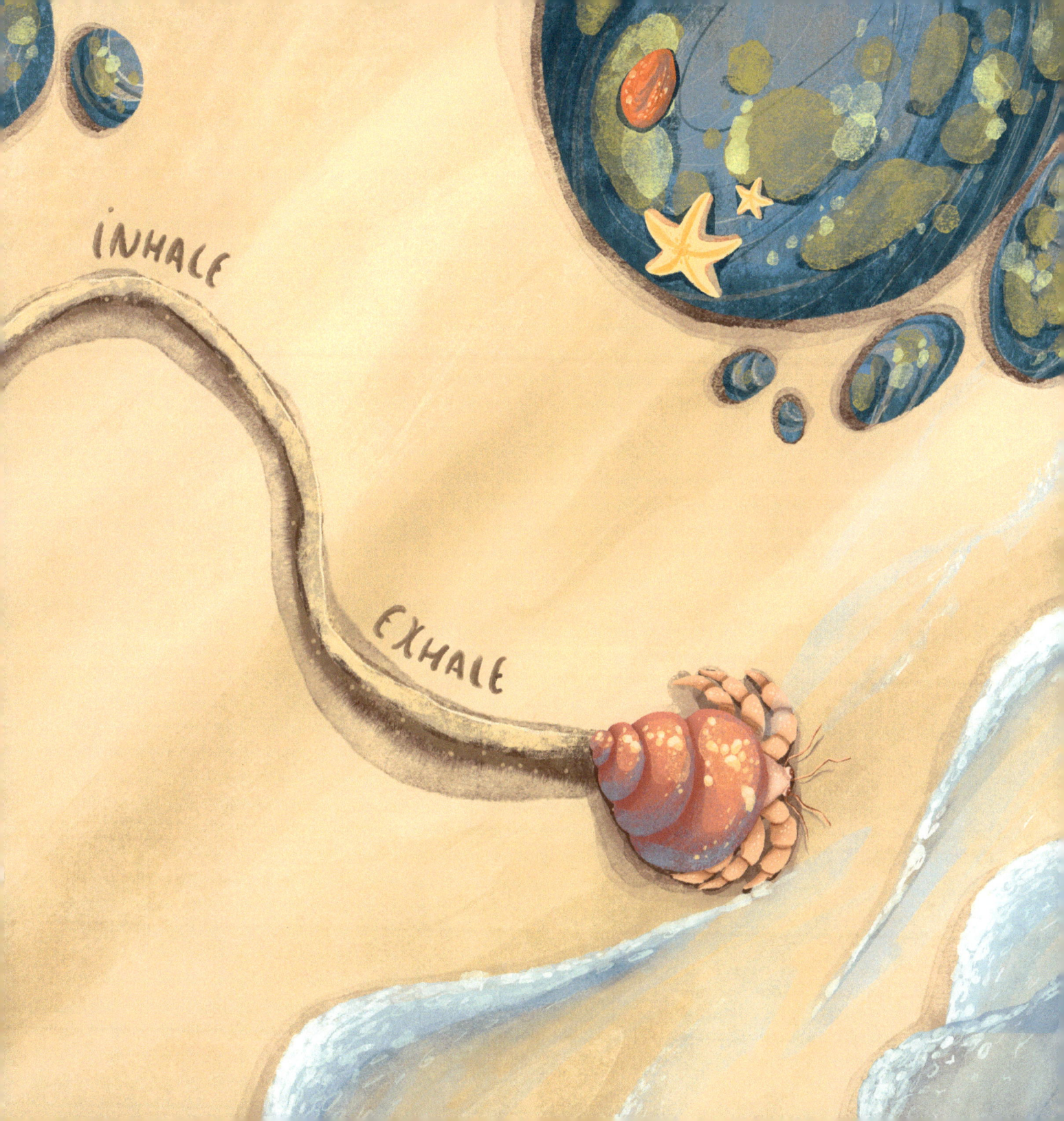

INHALE

EXHALE

Winnie,
Watching you run along the seaside inspired
me to write this book for you.
Keep shining bright.

By The Seaside

Written by Gretel Louise
Illustrated by Olena Kyrychenko

Copyright © 2025 Gretel Louise

All rights reserved. No part of this book may be reproduced
in any manner whatsoever without prior written permission
of the publisher.

First Printing, 2025

Published by Holistic Outcomes
www.holisticoutcomes.com.au

ISBN 978-1-7641112-0-1 Hardcover
ISBN 978-1-7641112-1-8 Paperback

NATIONAL LIBRARY OF AUSTRALIA

**A catalogue record for this
book is available from the
National Library of Australia.**

BY THE
SEASIDE

written by

GRETEL
LOUISE

illustrated by

OLENA
KYRYCHENKO

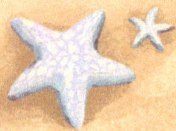

By the seaside is where I go,
to feel the warm sunshine and soft winds blow.

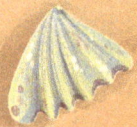

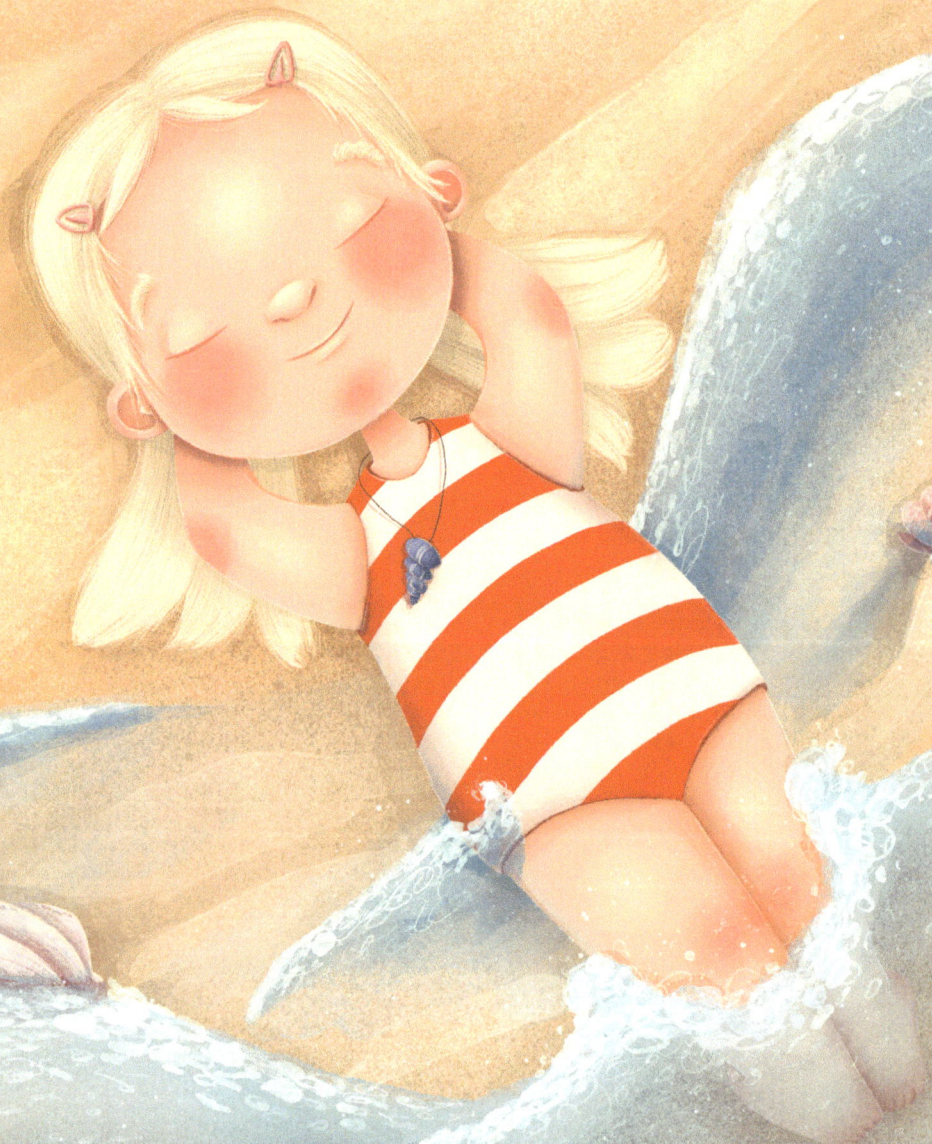

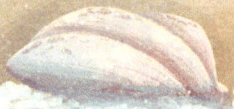

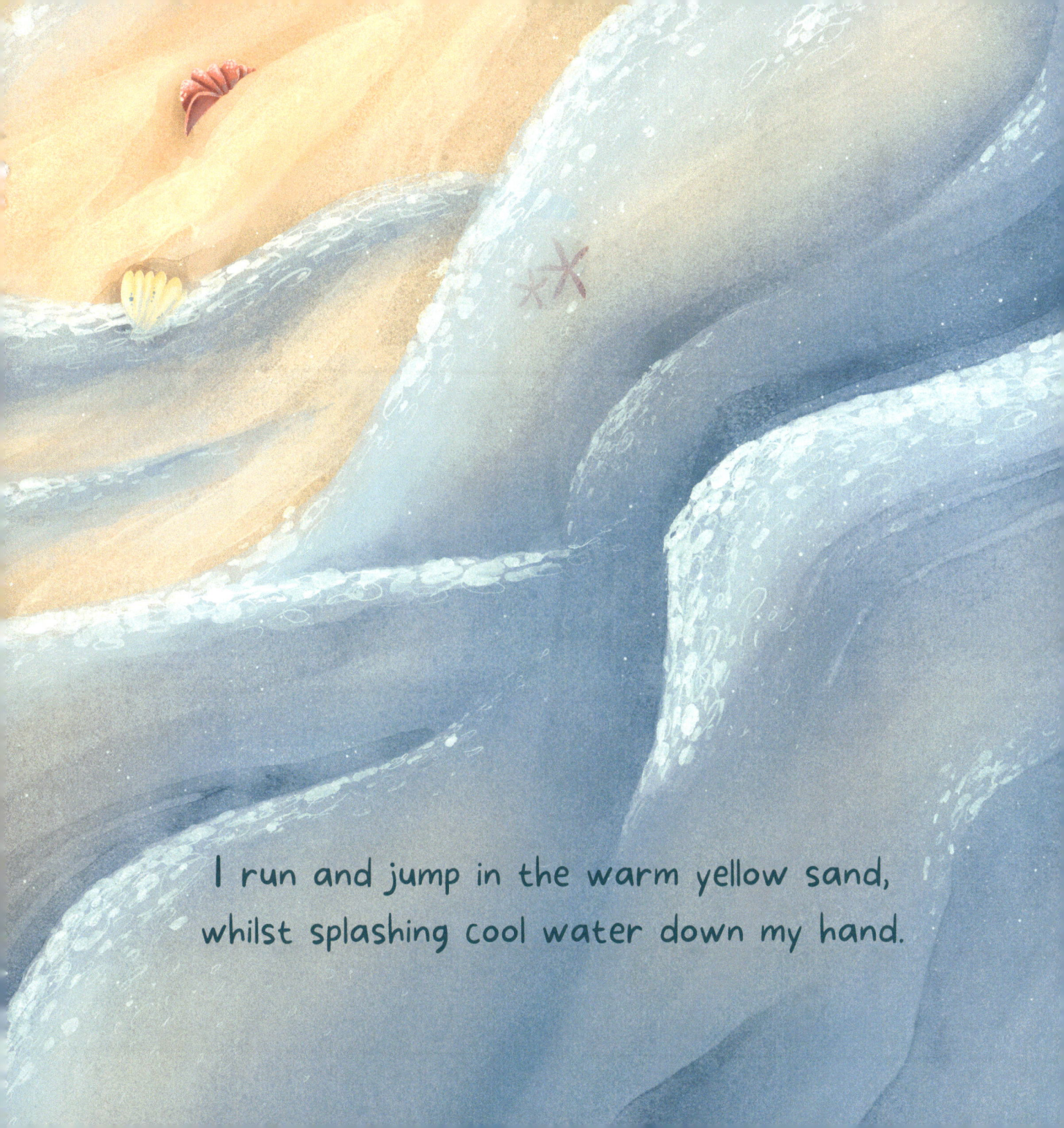

I run and jump in the warm yellow sand,
whilst splashing cool water down my hand.

I sit on the beach and think of things.
Cats, dogs and birds that sing.

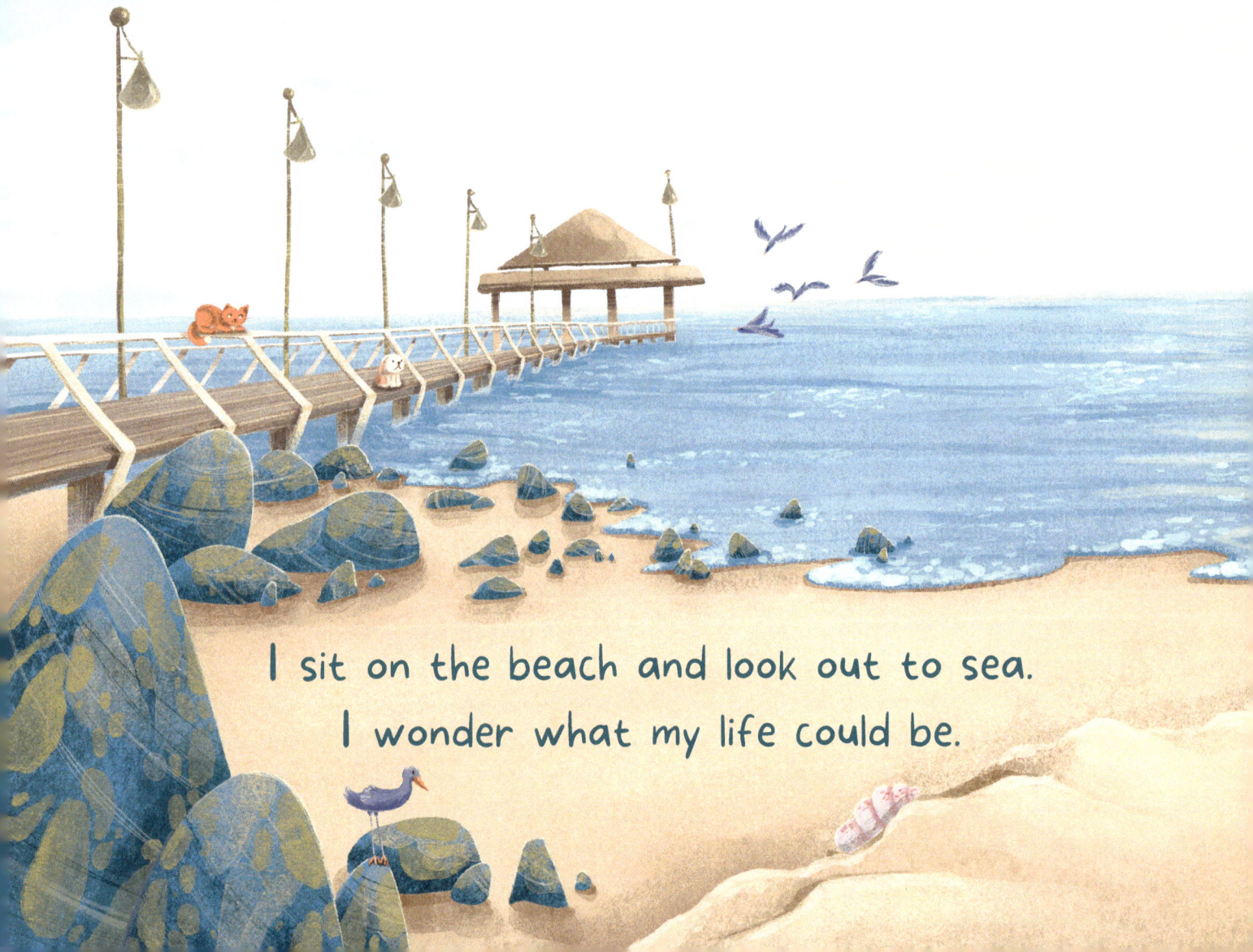

I sit on the beach and look out to sea.
I wonder what my life could be.

By the seaside is where I go,
when my heart and mind are feeling low.

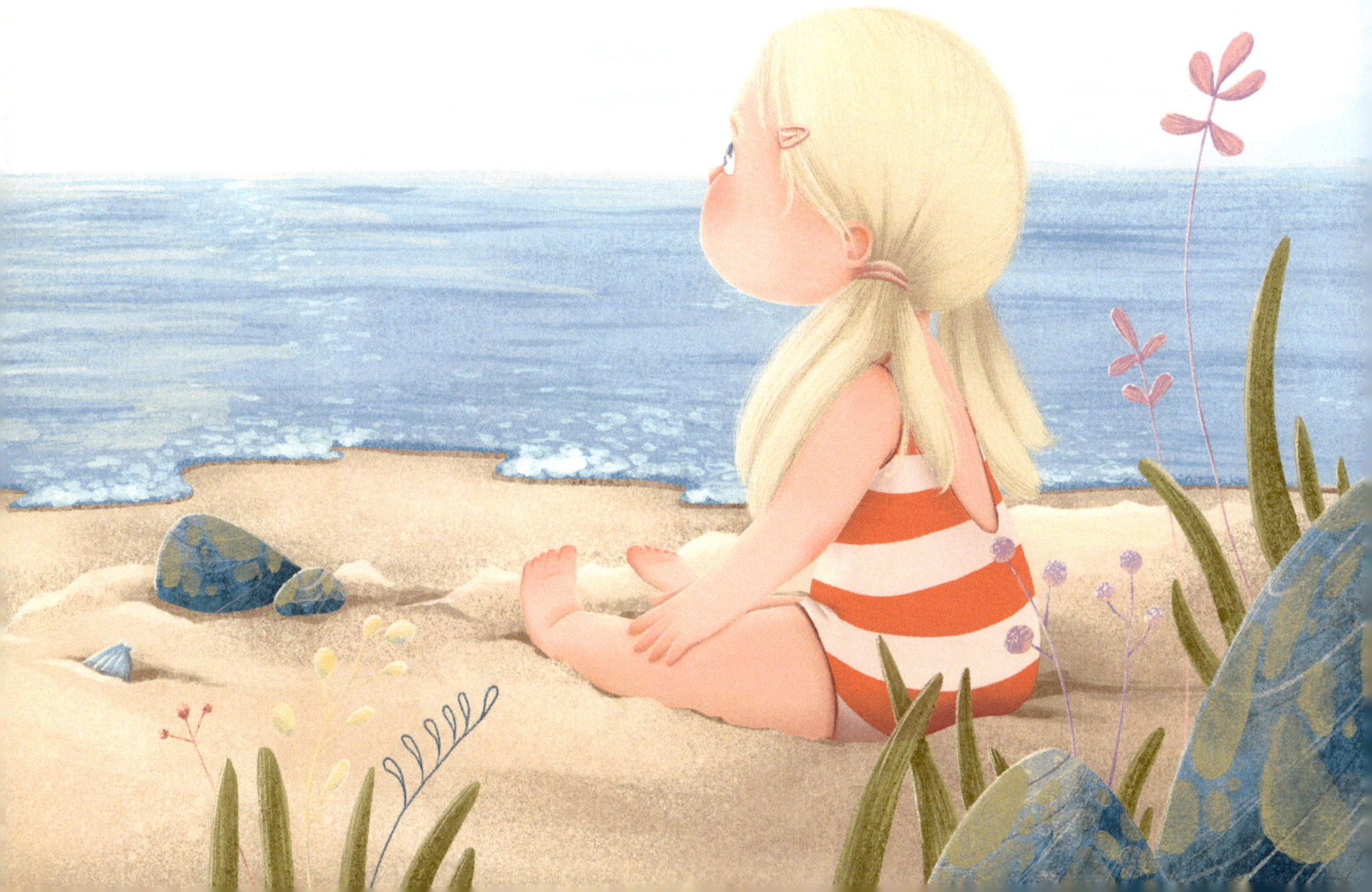

When you've had a bad day,
and things haven't gone your way...
it's time to head outside,
and keep those feelings at bay.

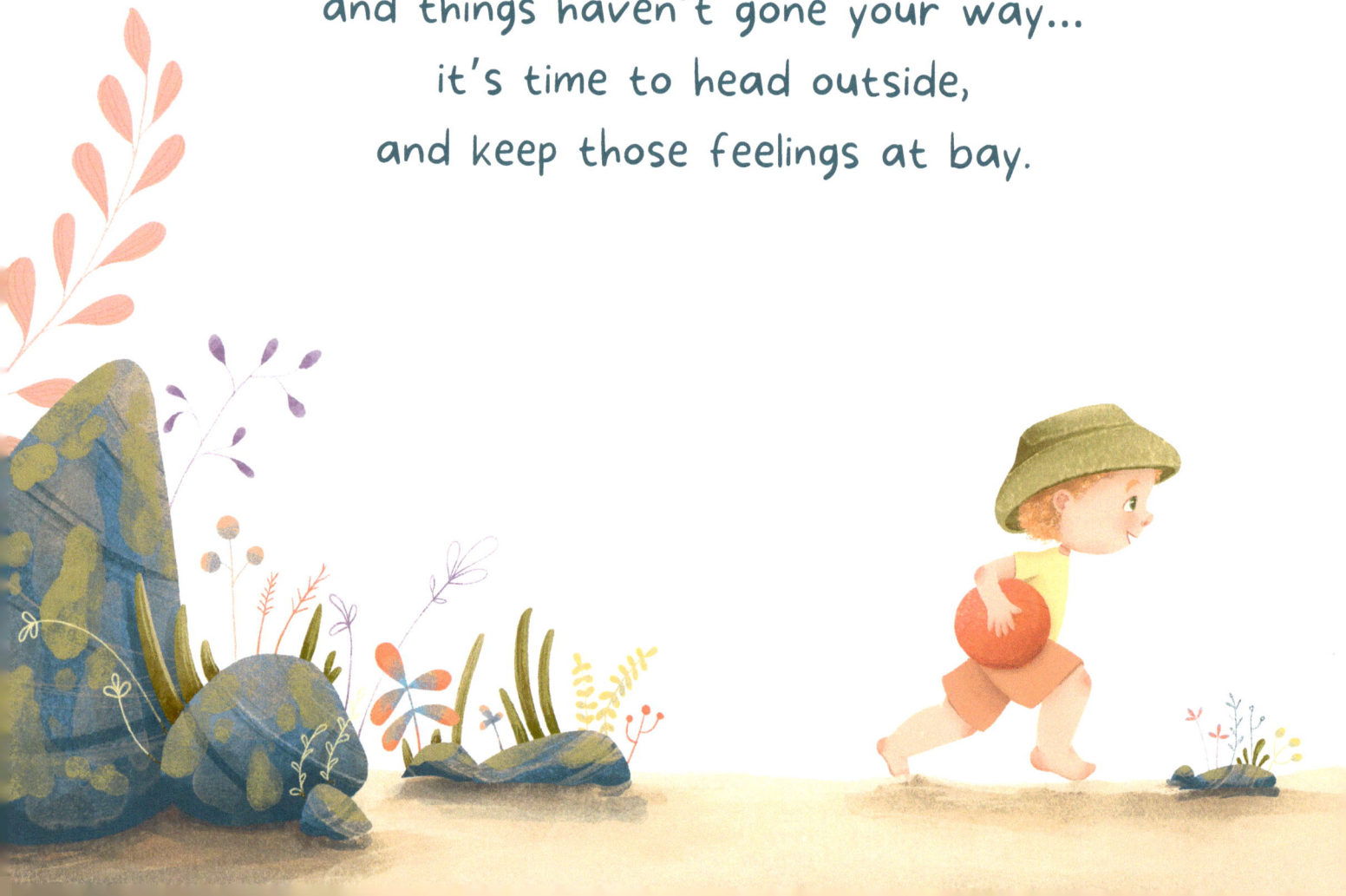

By the sea is where I feel free...
I love it by the water,
it's my favourite place to be.

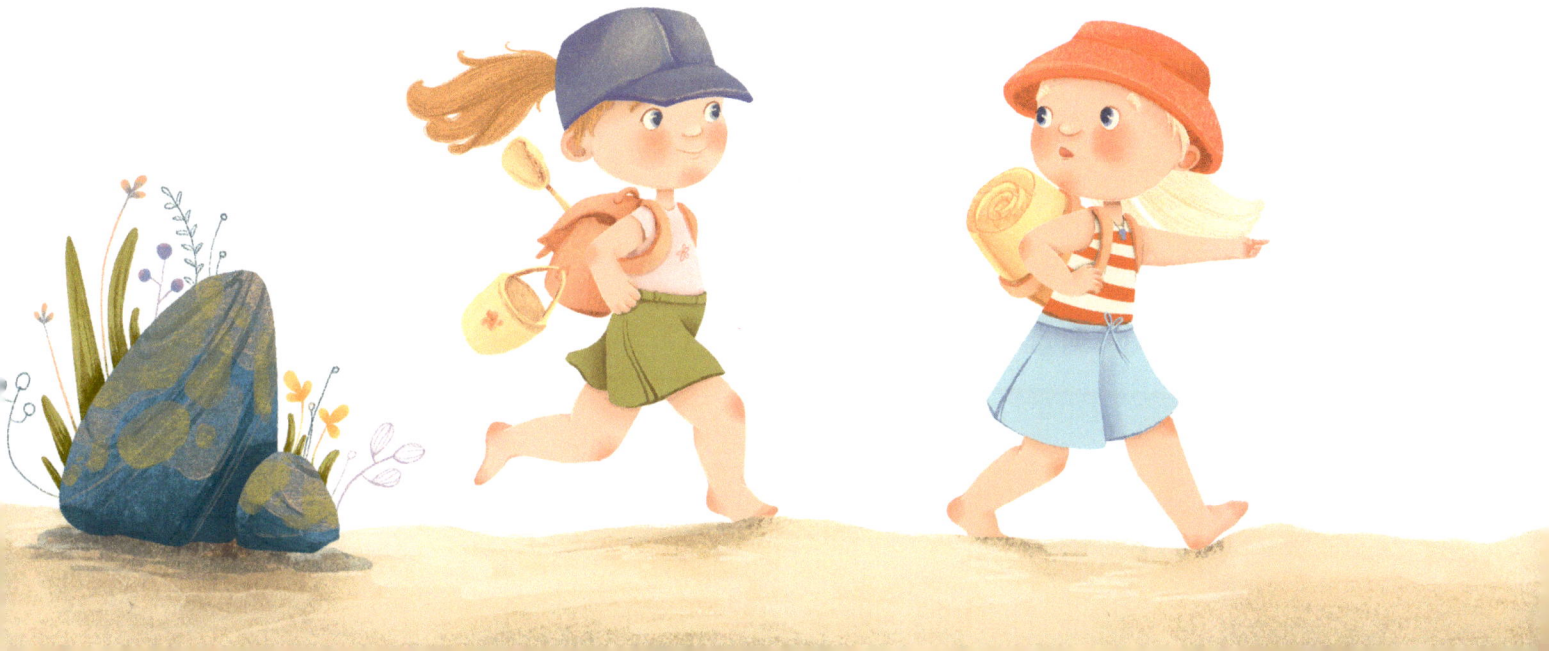

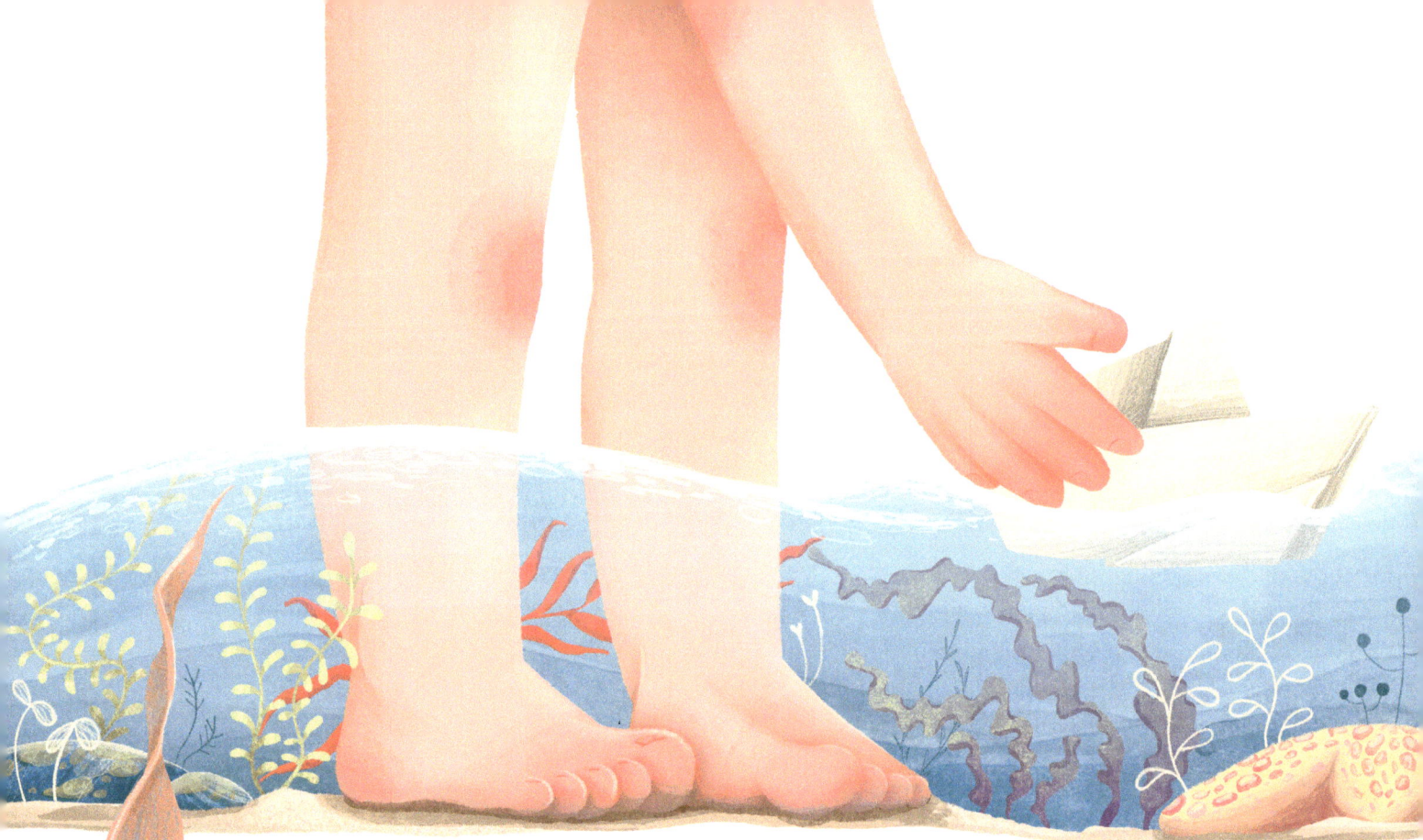

By the seaside is where I go,
to calm my heavy feelings,
and not let them grow.

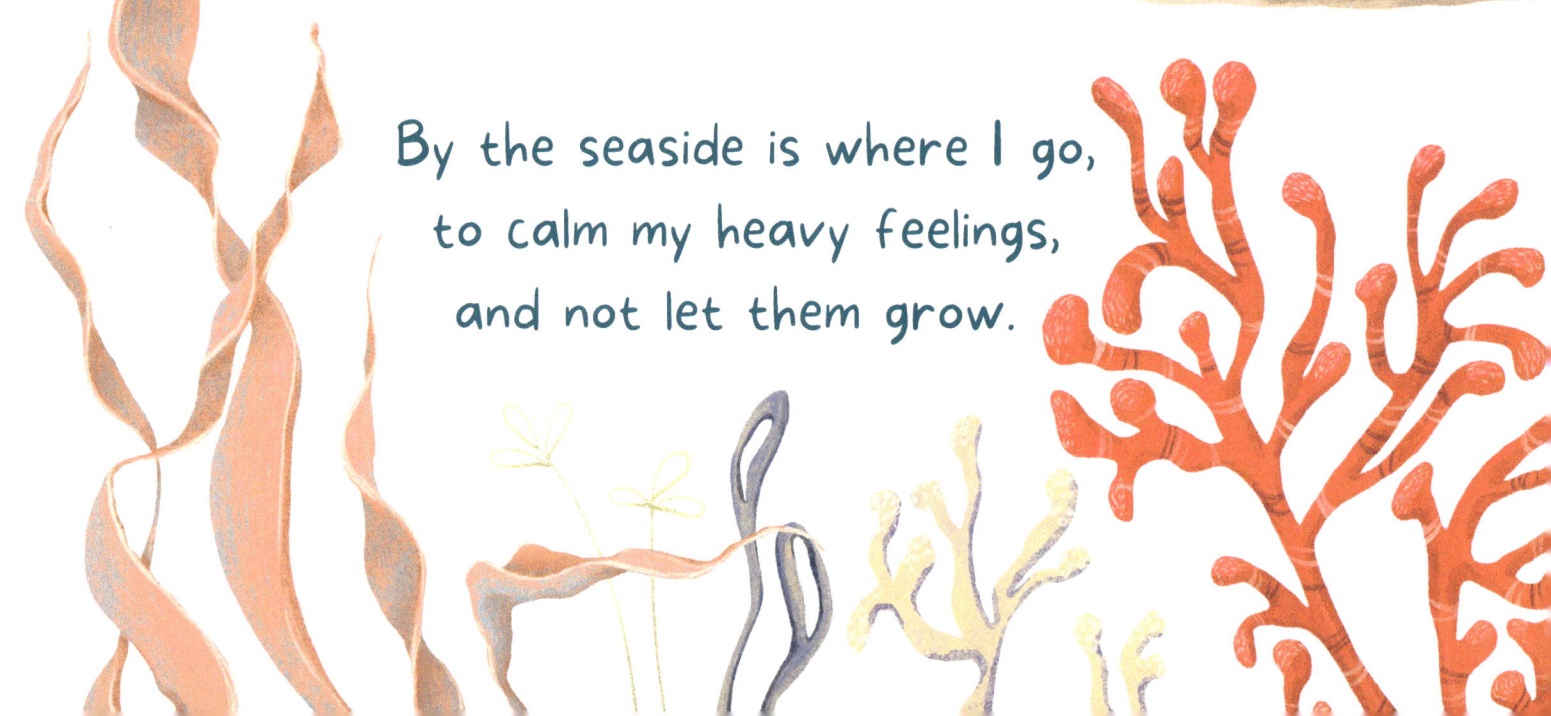

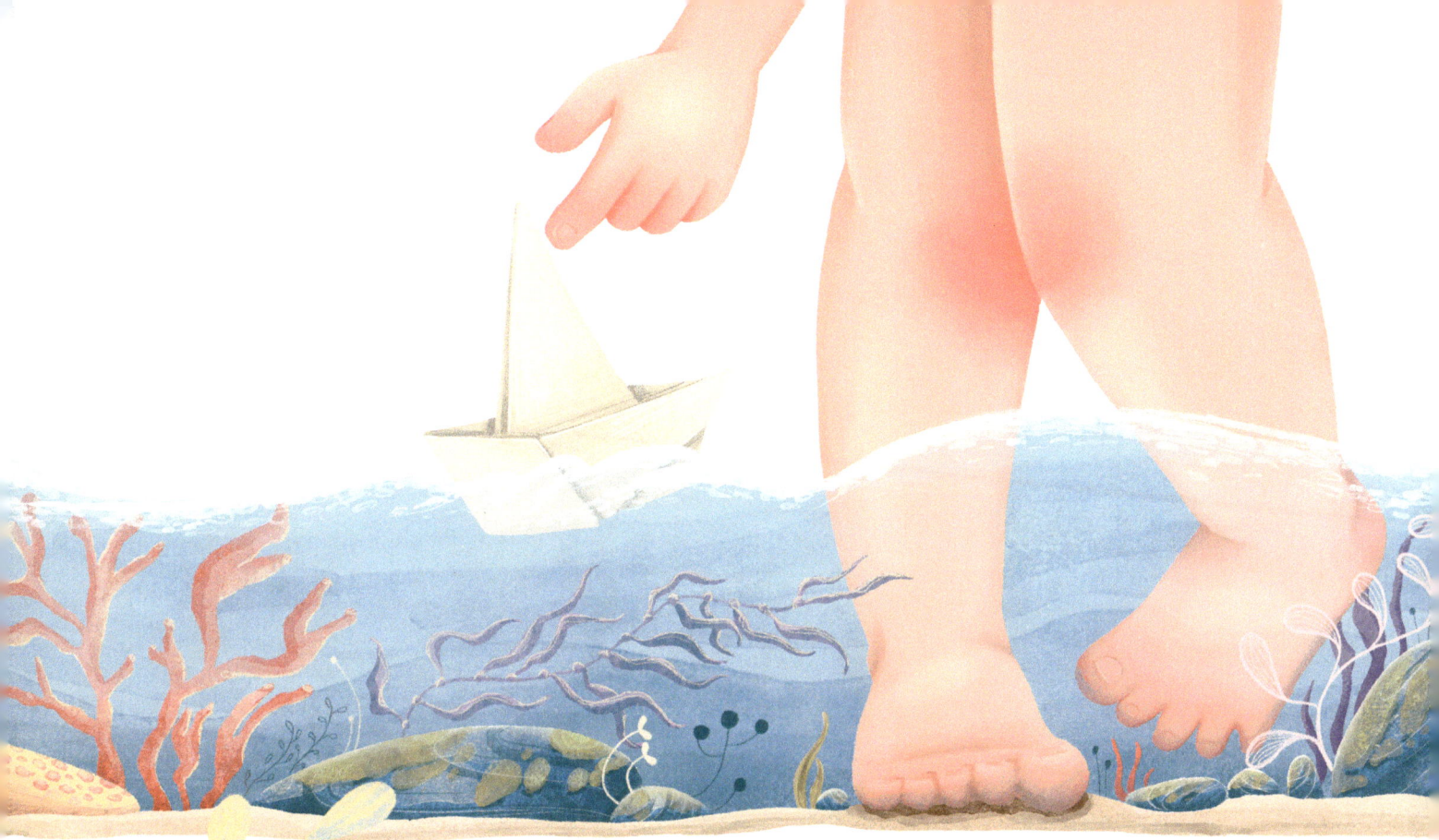

Being in nature helps calm my mind,
I love the seaside
as it helps me find.....

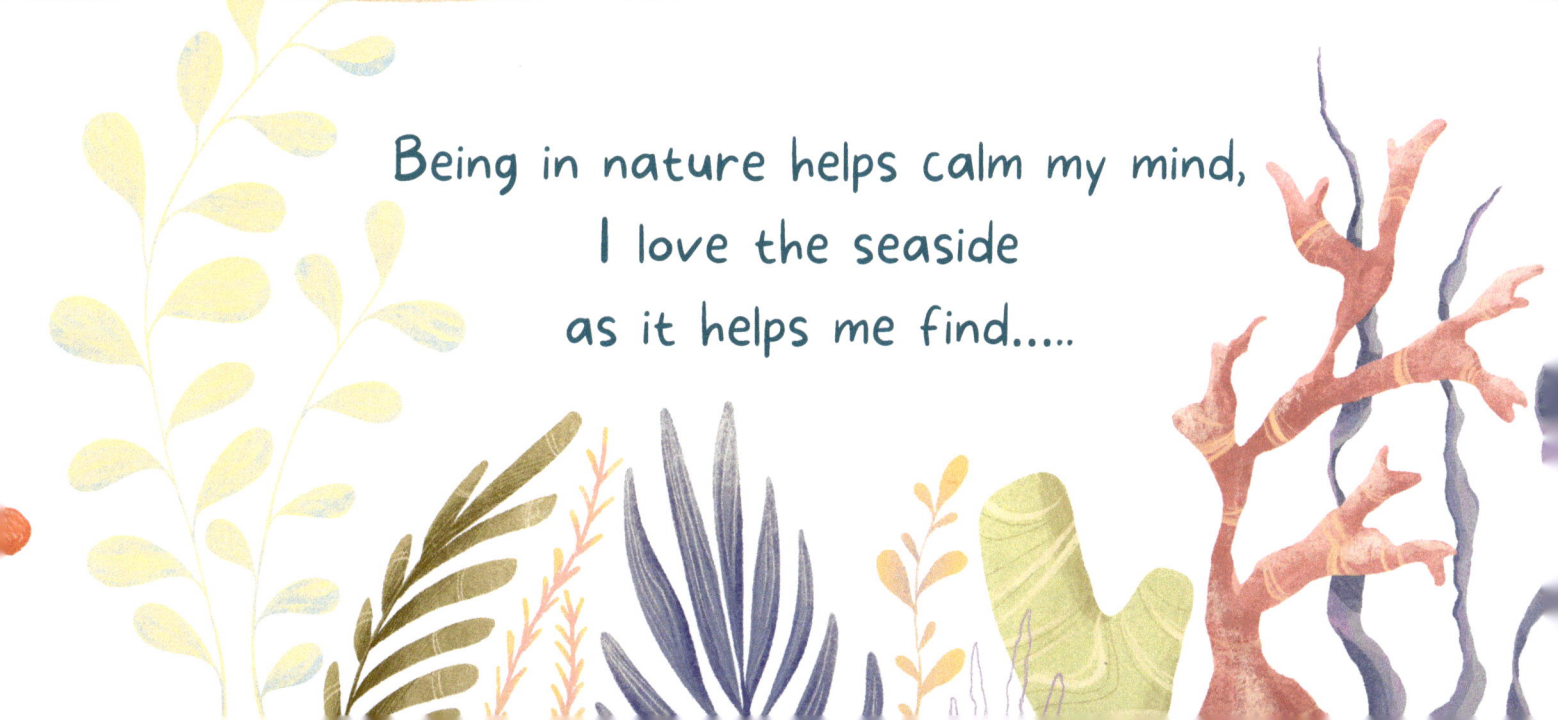

A WAY...

to SHAKE...

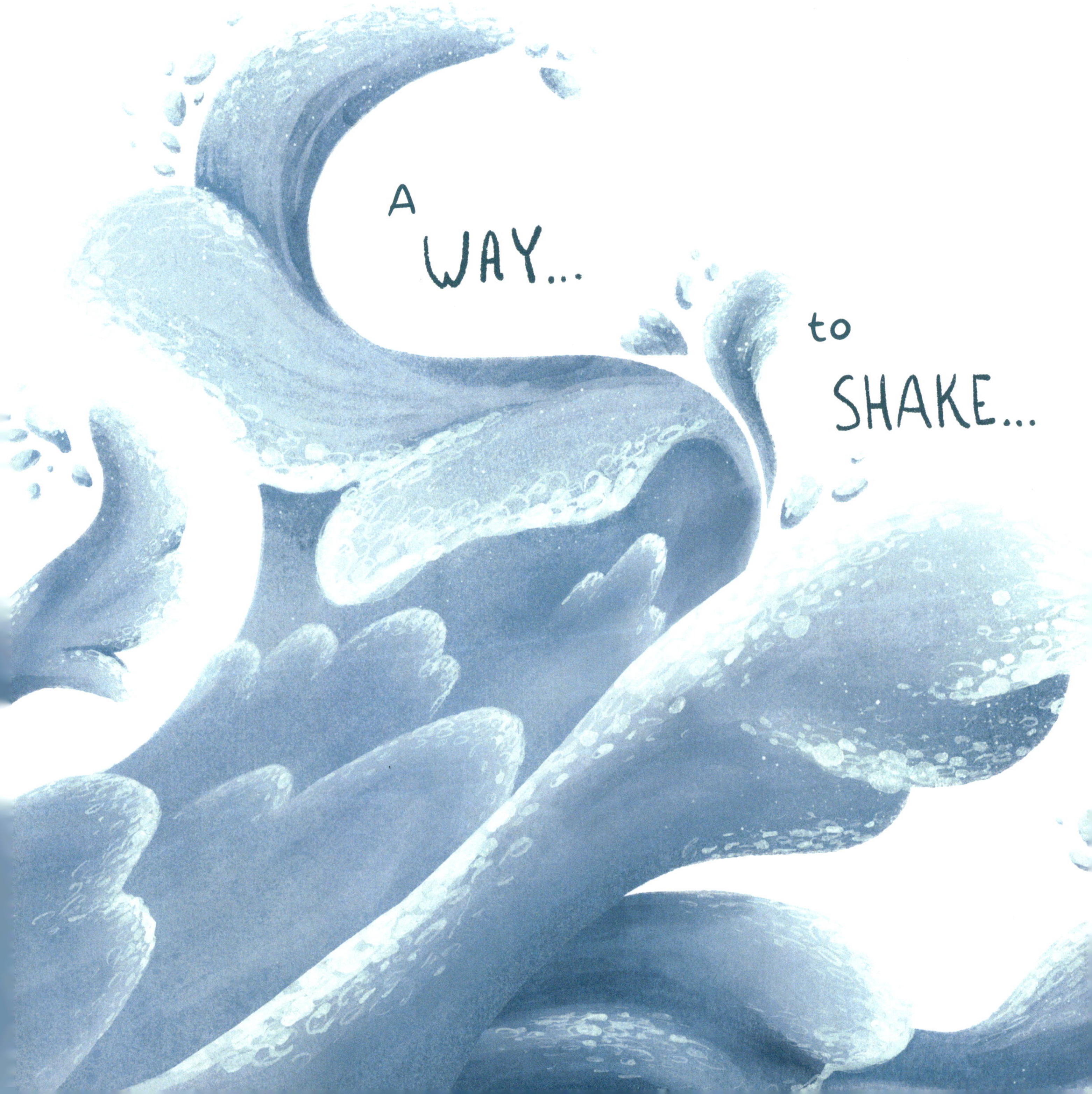

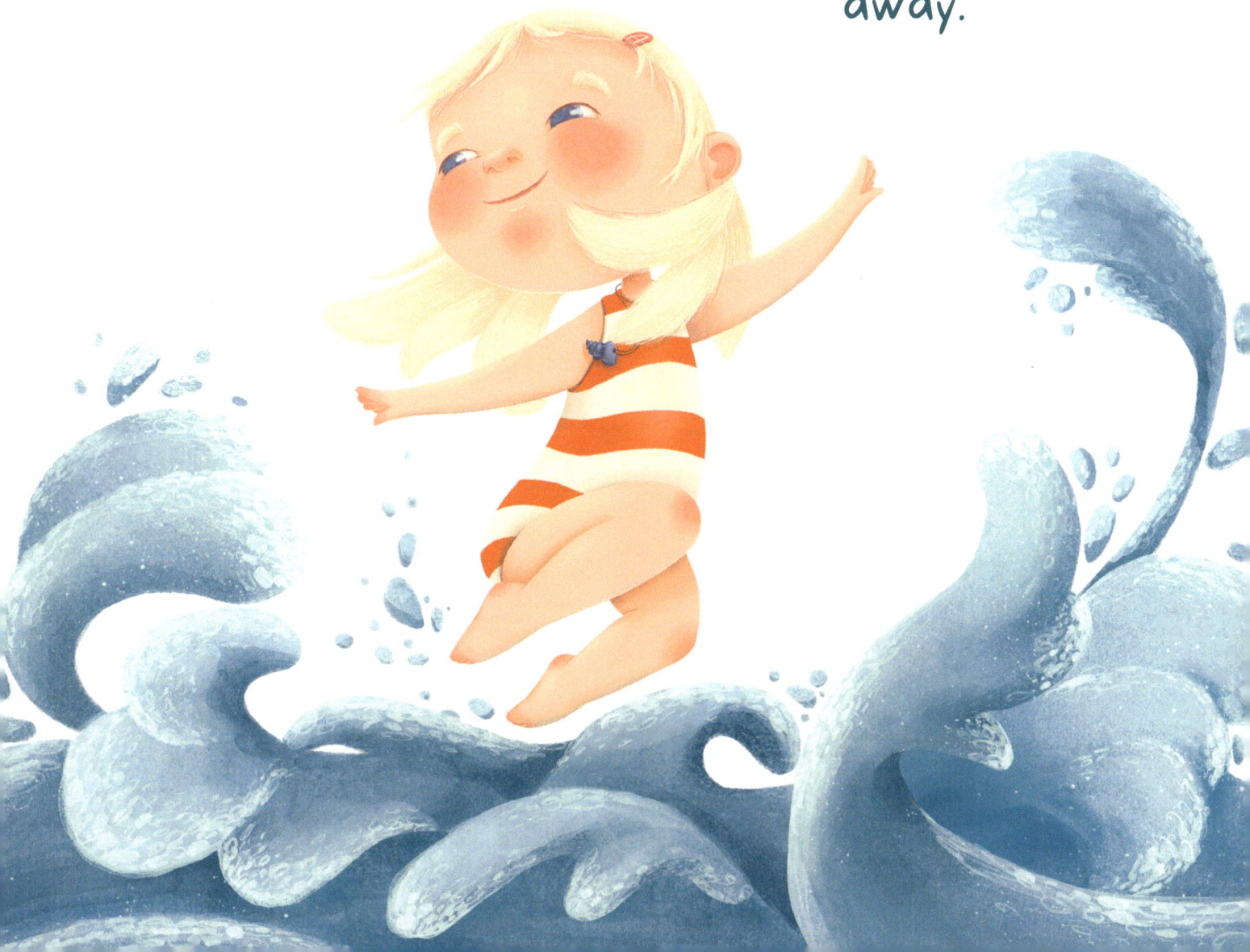

those

WORRIES...

away.

By the seaside is where I go...
to help ground my thoughts,
and make them nice and slow.

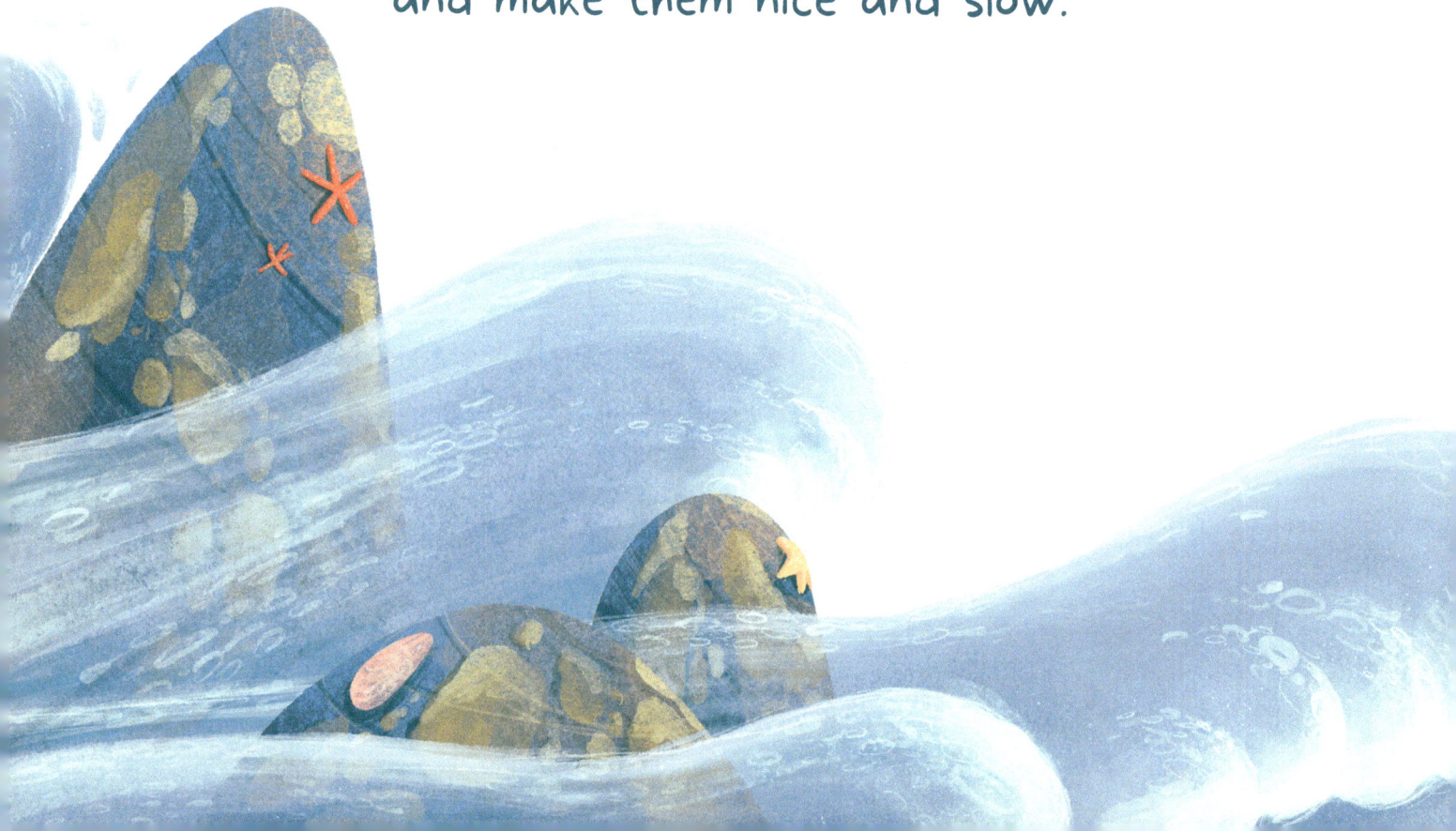

I take a deep breath through my nose,

and suddenly.....

it feels like all my troubles froze.

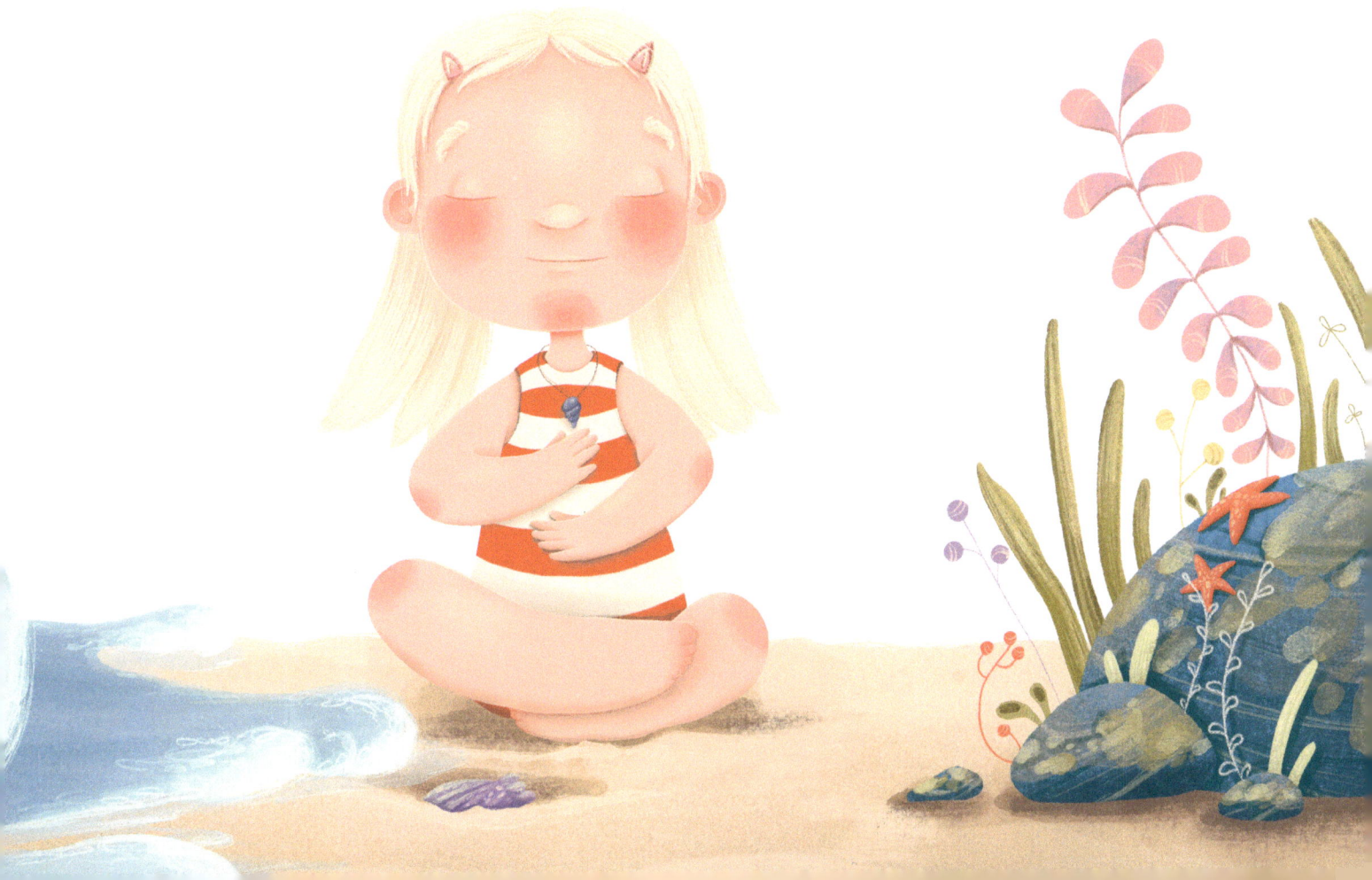

As the waves roll in,
I breathe through my nose,

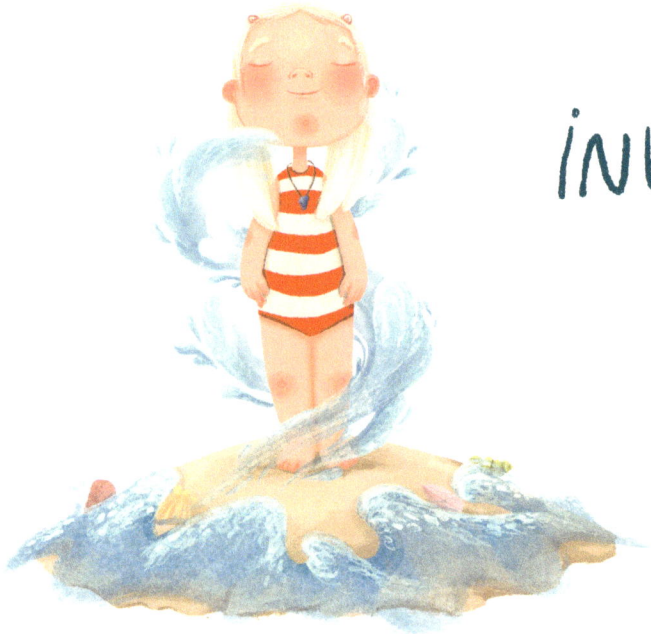

INHALE...

EXHALE,

and out the air goes.

As I breathe out, I feel so free...
as all my worries drift out to sea.

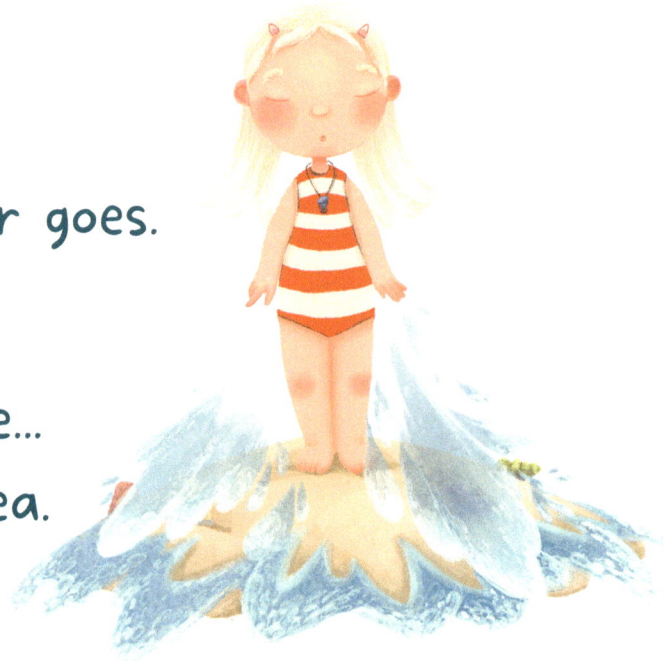

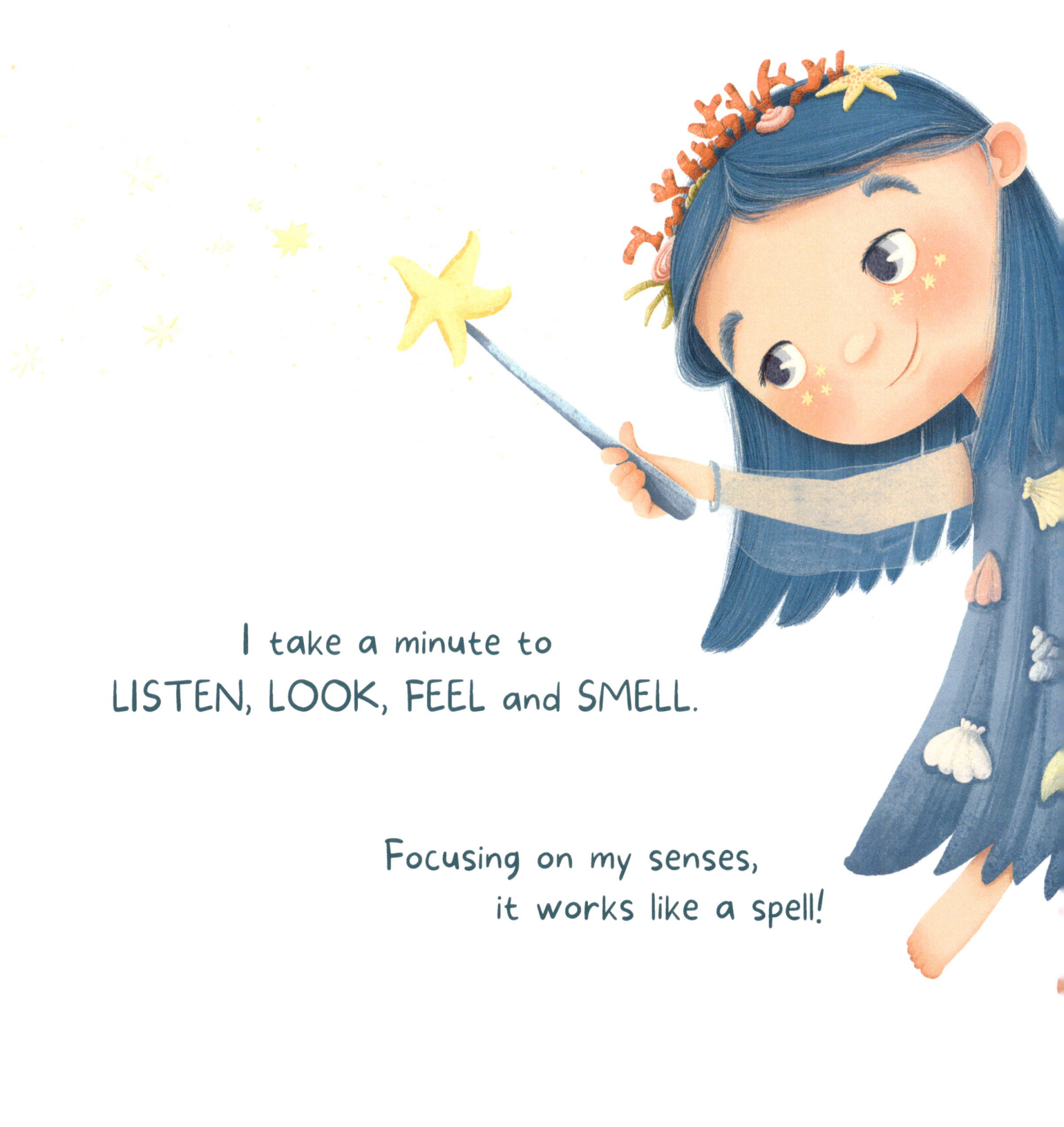

I take a minute to
LISTEN, LOOK, FEEL and SMELL.

Focusing on my senses,
it works like a spell!

I LISTEN
with my ears to hear,

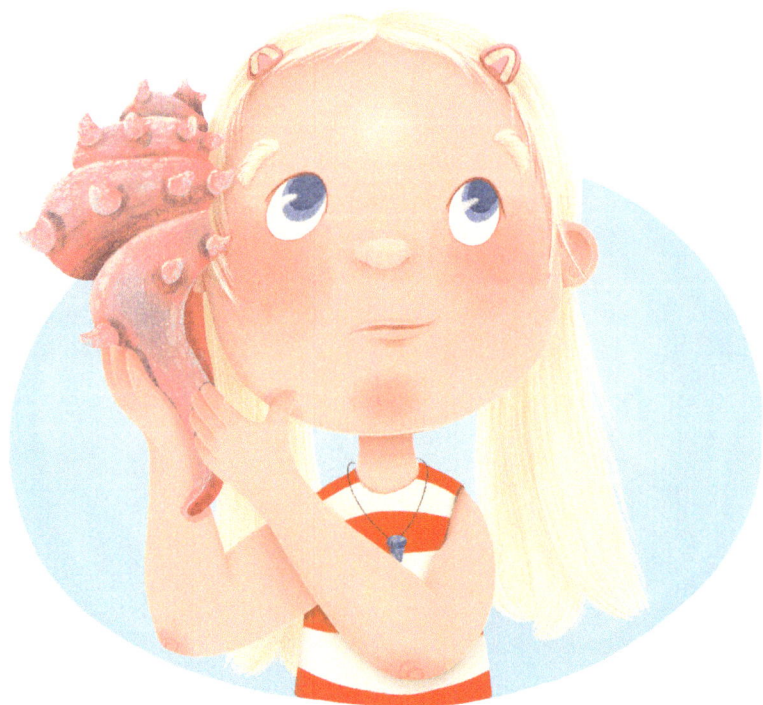

LOOK
with my eyes at things near.

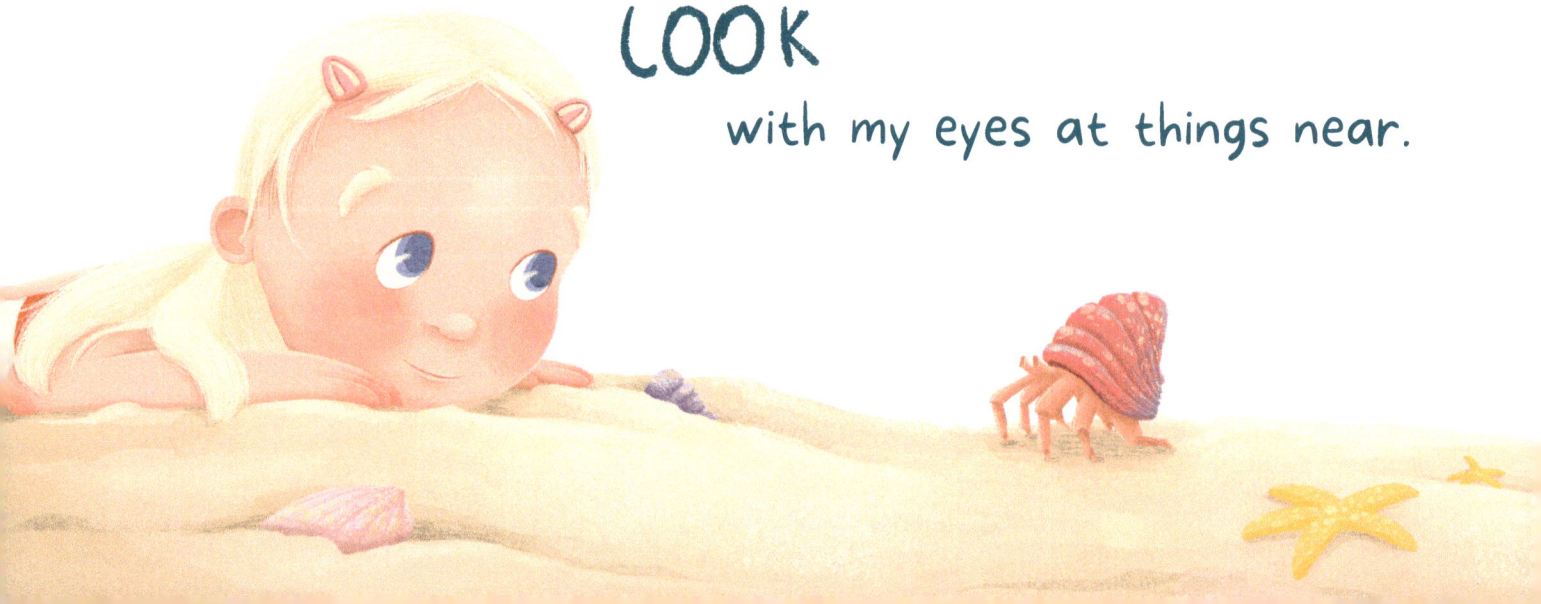

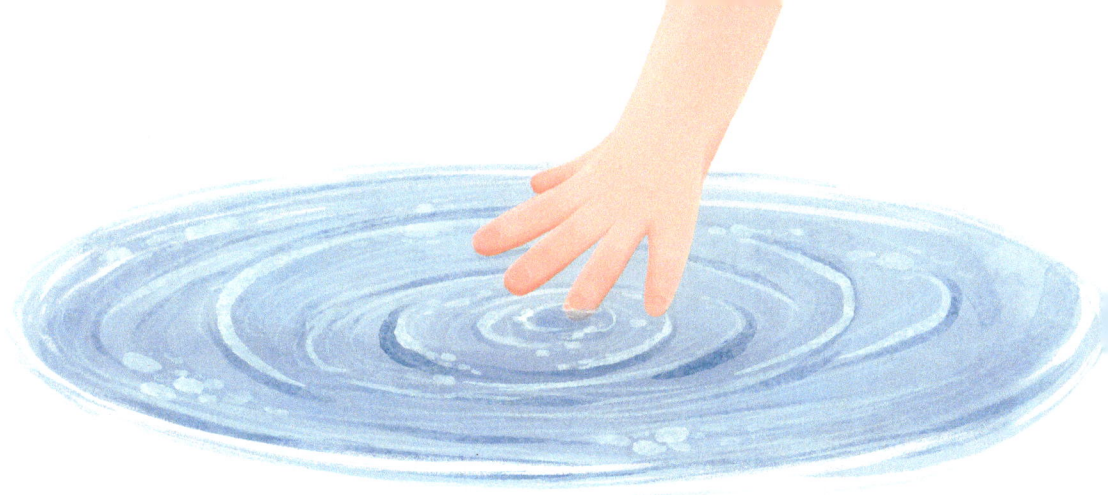

FEEL with my body to touch,

and SMELL the scents I enjoy so much.

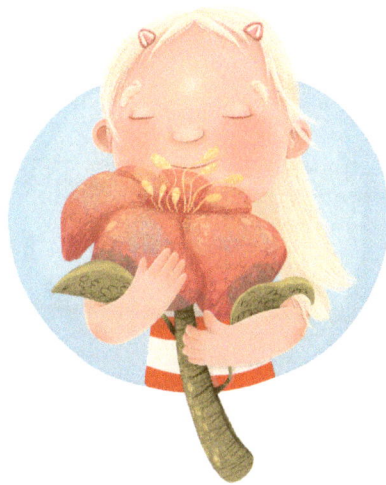

I HEAR the waves crashing down,
and the cars passing through town.

I SEE the boats sailing out to sea,
and the birds flying above me.

I FEEL the sand beneath my feet,
and the sun shining with heat.

I SMELL the salt that fills the air,
and a sausage sizzle drifting everywhere.

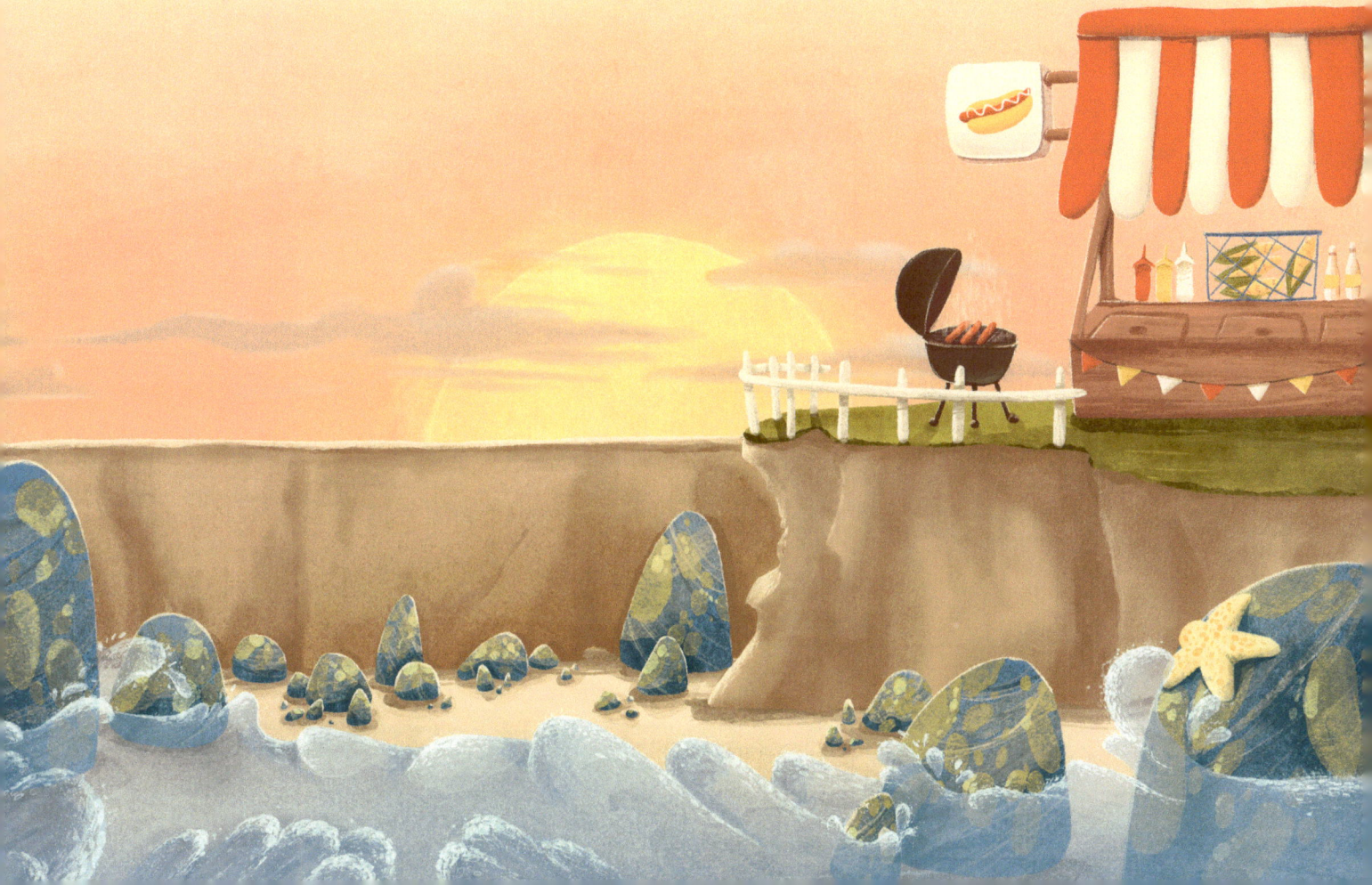

Being outside
helps ground my senses.

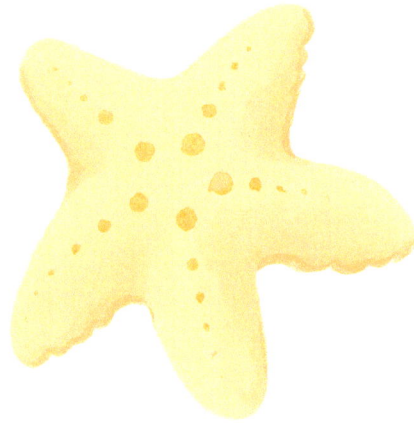

I love being outdoors,
it's one of our greatest defences.

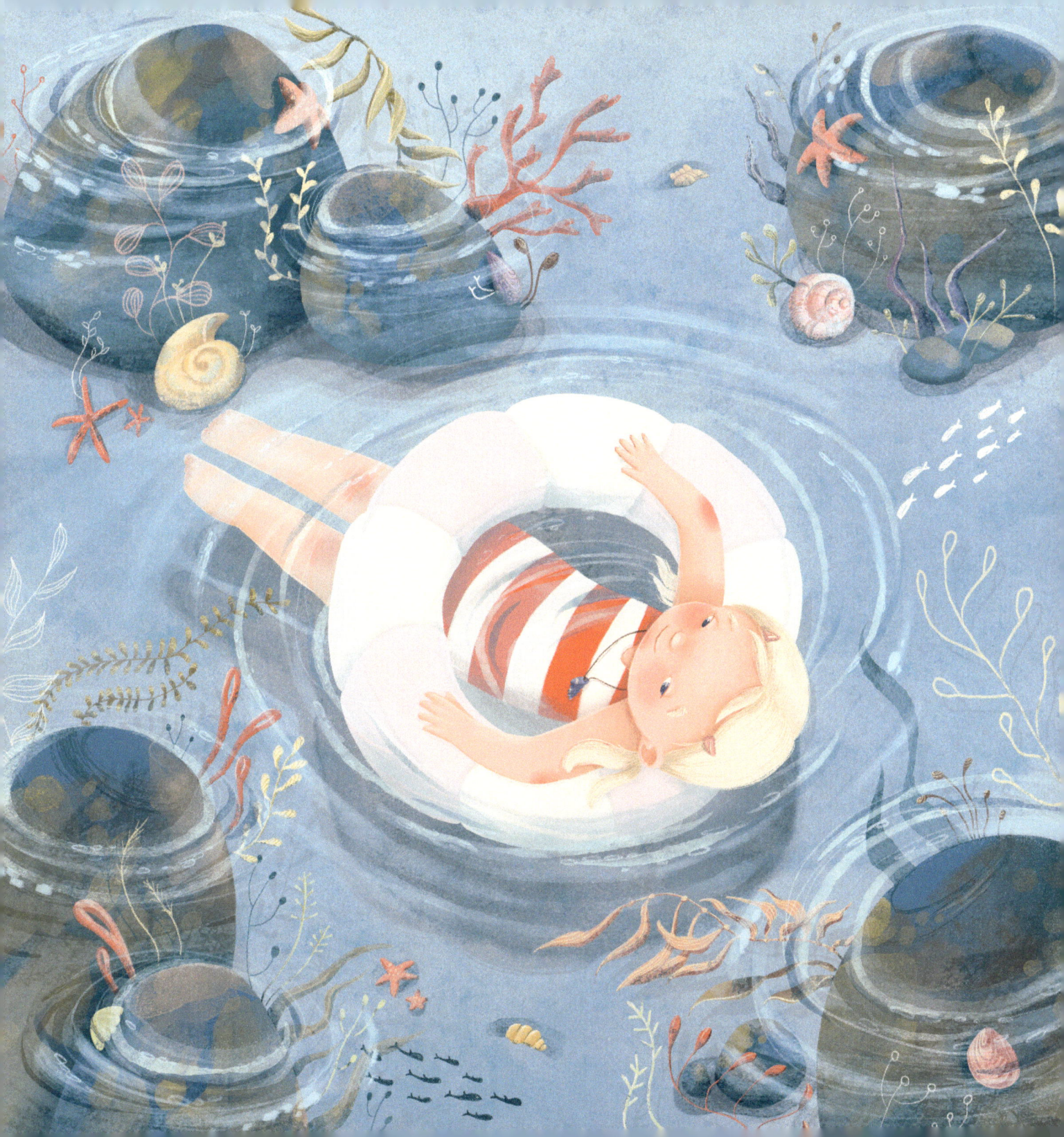

When your mind is feeling busy,
or your heart is feeling low...

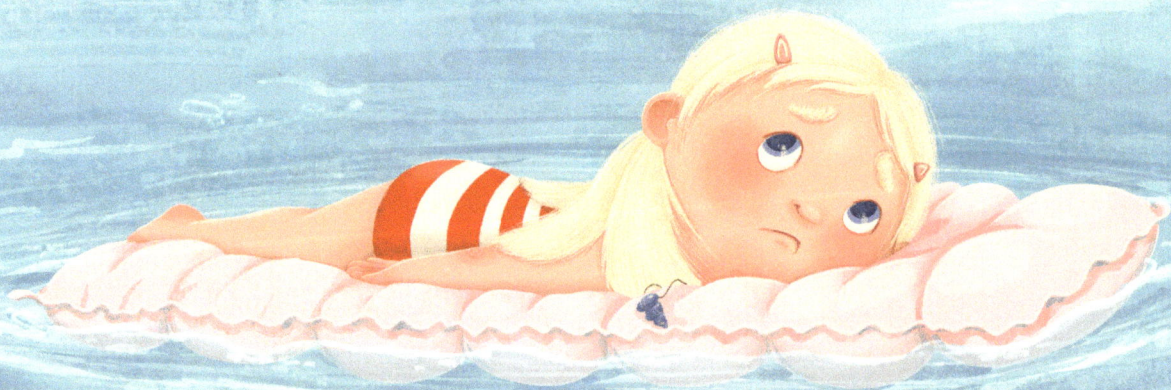

Get your body moving,
and go with the flow.

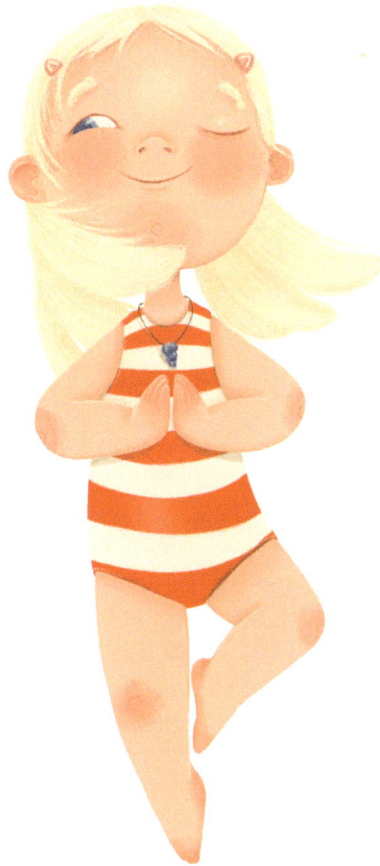

I can dance and jump,
to get out of my slump.

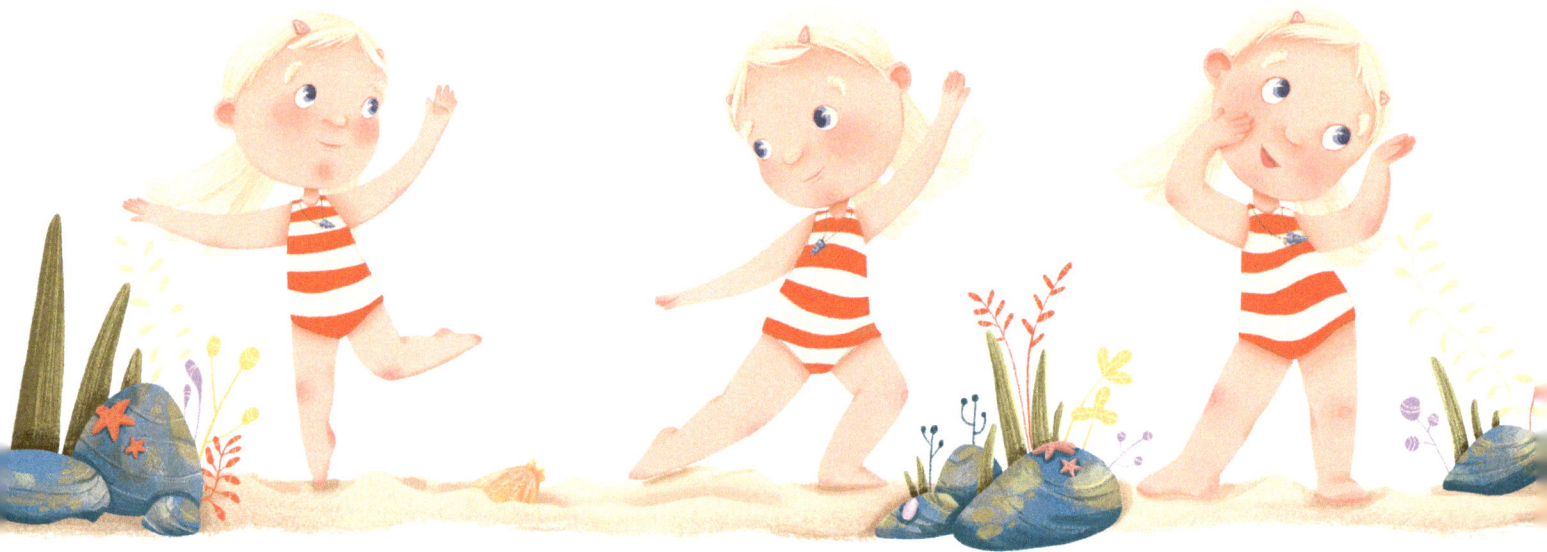

I can move and groove,
to improve my mood.

I can leap and soar,
to let my spirit explore.

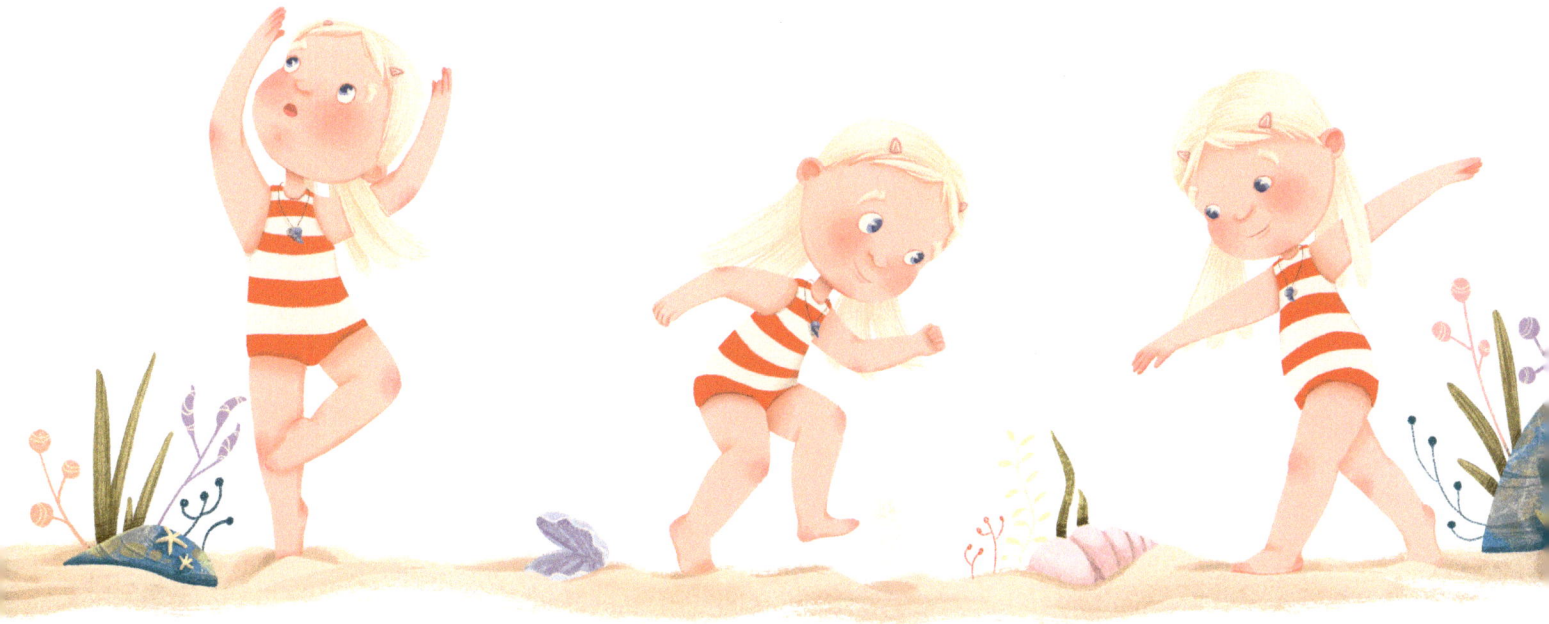

I can twist and sway,
to brighten my day.

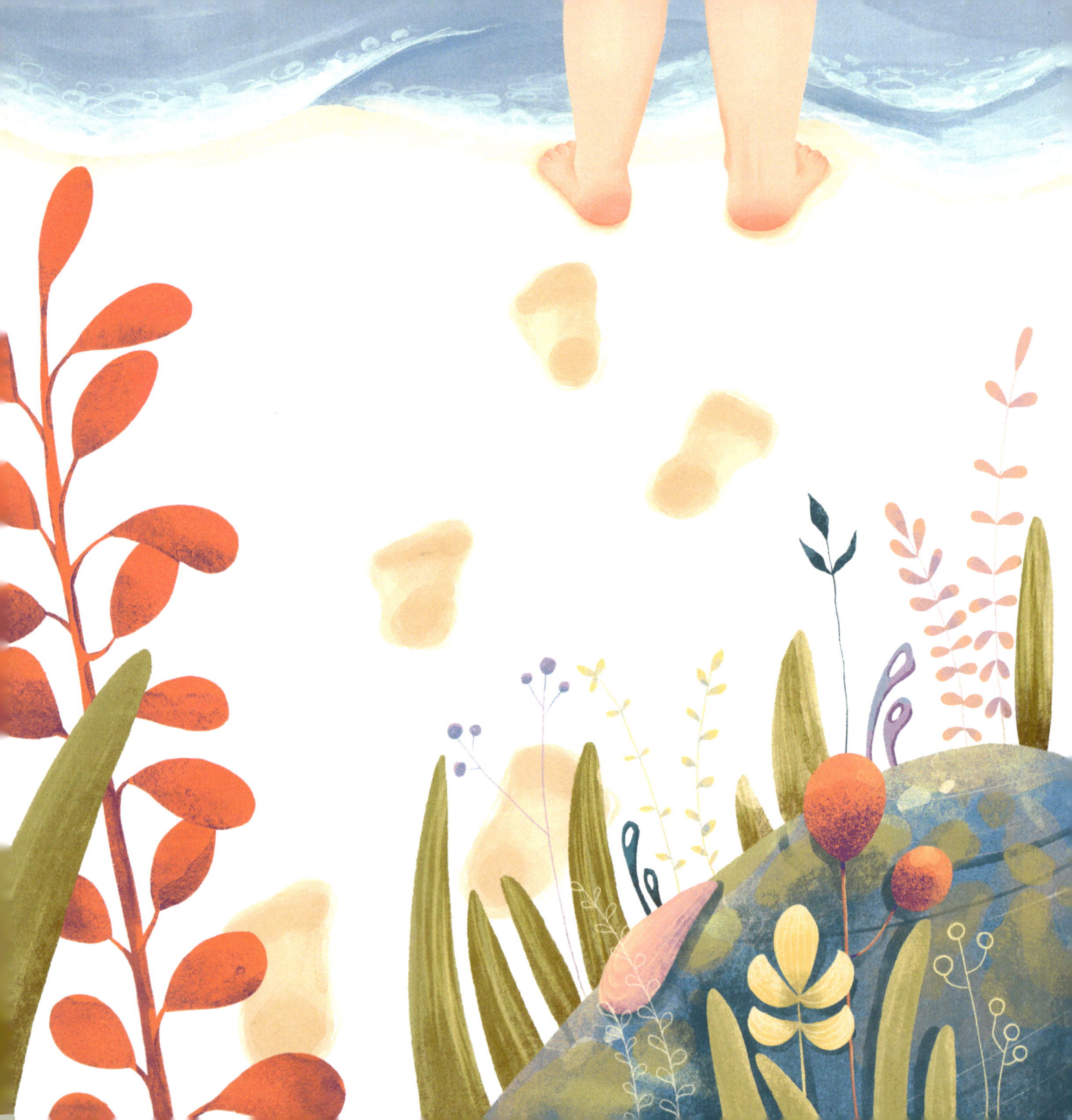

When my feet touch the sand,
it helps me understand...

that with each step I take,
I find my way...

to enjoy a bright, cheerful
and happy day.

By the seaside is where I go...

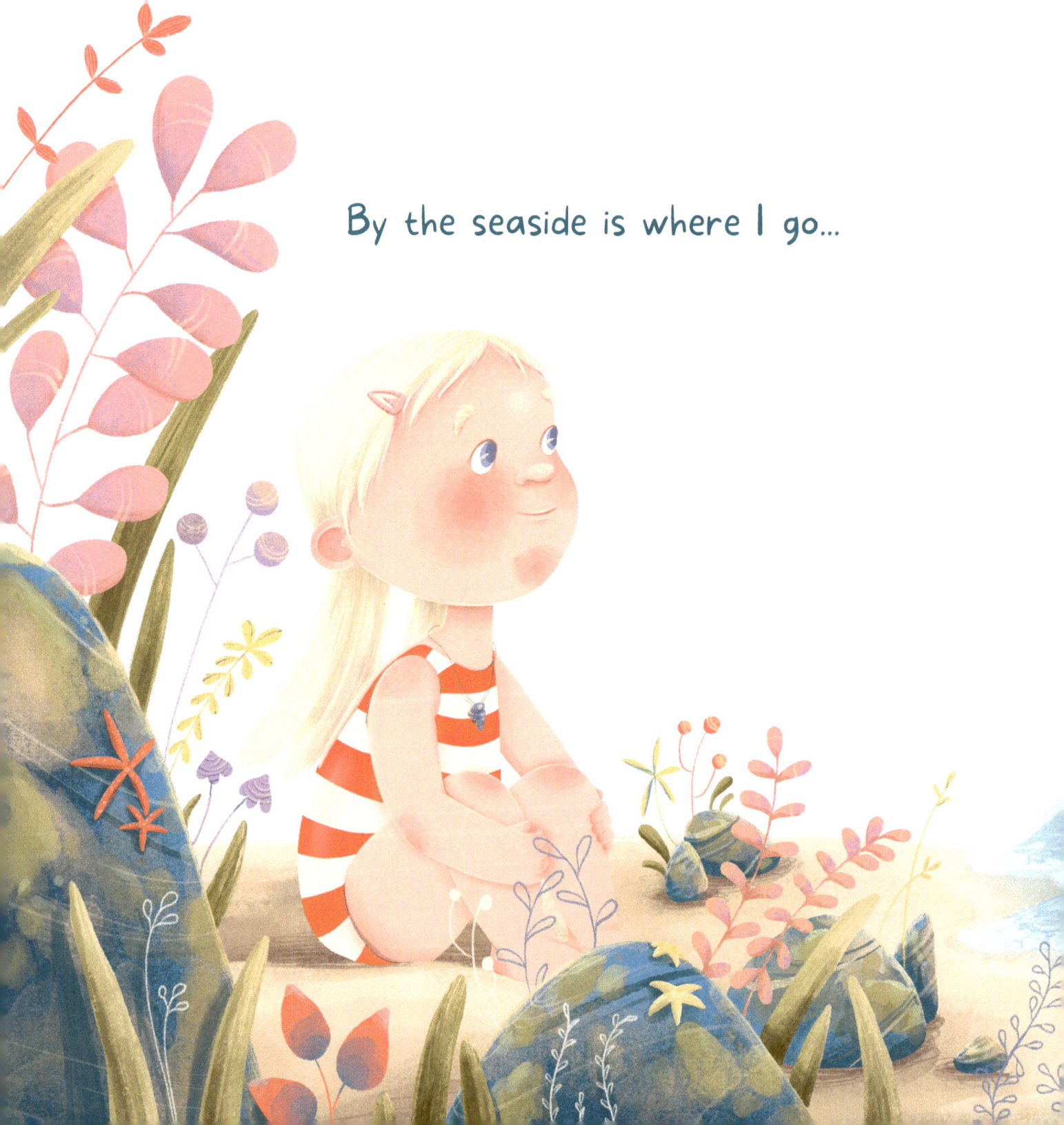

to calm my mind and my body,

from my head to my toes.

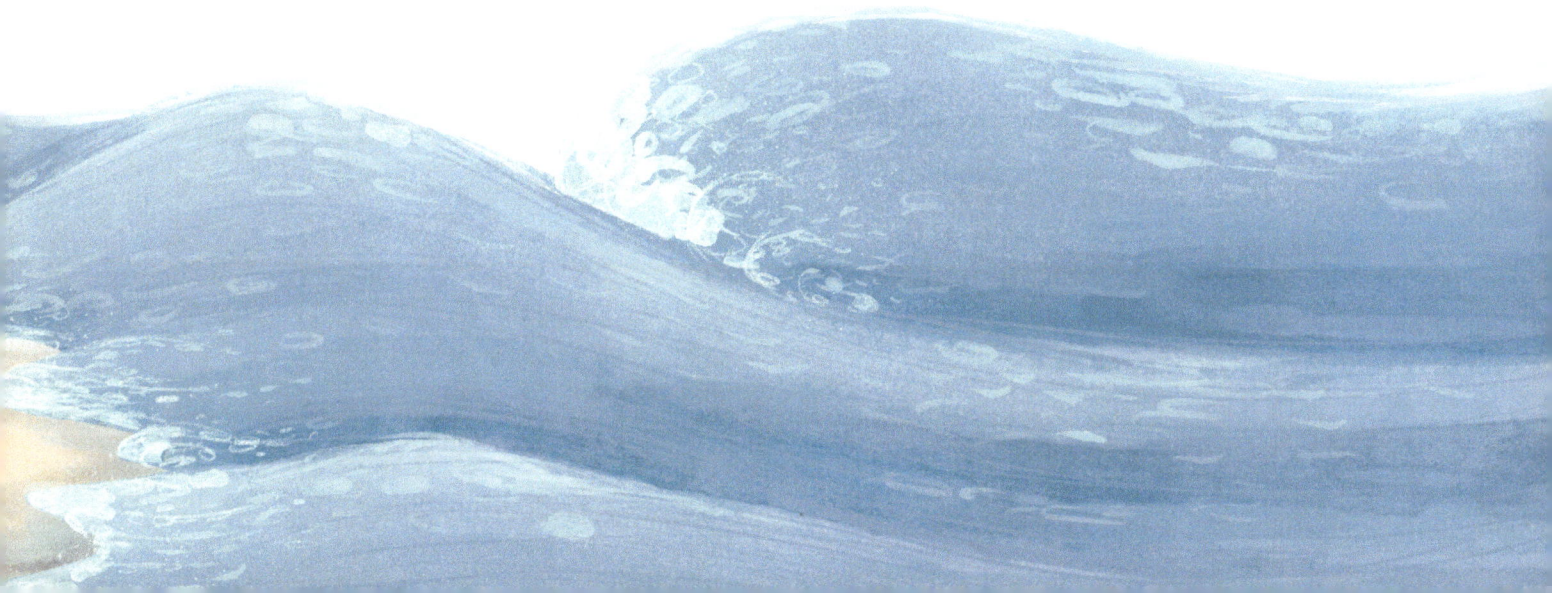

www.ingramcontent.com/pod-product-compliance
Lightning Source LLC
Chambersburg PA
CBHW041547260326
41914CB00016B/1572